DDJ PUBLISHING

THE PERFECT GOLF SWING IN MINUTES

THE BEST EVER METHOD, BEGINNER OR PRO FOR CONTROL, ACCURACY, FEEL, CONSISTENCY, AND EFFORTLESS POWER. THE SECRET, MAGIC MOVE IN ONE SIMPLE LESSON. DRILL, REPEAT, AND ALWAYS HIT GREAT SHOTS.

Contents

1

Introduction

A ll golfers would like to have a good dependable golf swing. At the very least they'd just like to be a respectable player. Why is this one goal so difficult to achieve, and why is it so challenging to do in a NATURAL, INSTINCTIVE way?

Well, the problem is that we actually need to be taught to swing the golf club in a more natural, instinctive way. With today's modern, more analytical swing methods and approaches, ironically, we have actually gone backwards in our learning progress.

Even with the advent of video instruction and scientific, bio mechanical models to help us, the golf swing remains a mystery to most. Even for those at the top of the game it can become more elusive than expected.

Whether it is the complex nature of this sometimes mechanical game or the methods of instruction gone wrong, statistics show over the last several decades that handicap averages have been getting worse for the golf population not better.

In this short book, I'm going to give you and hopefully even enlighten you to the incredibly simple and powerful way of learning to swing a golf club. It is a more natural, instinctive, and effective way. It is so user-friendly and relatively effortless, that you might read this short book quickly on the range or just before a round and begin using your near perfect swing with amazing results.

2

Is There a Single Secret to Golf?

Well, the answer could be yes and no. To put it more bluntly, no, because there are a lot of aspects to the game that we are not even addressing, but as far as the golf swing goes the answer gets a bit more positive.

Good or bad, it's the golf swing that everyone generally loves and admires the most, that creates the thrill for the audience, but that baffles most if not all players at times. With that in mind, this may be the closest thing there is to a best, single secret of the golf swing.

Since you are unique as an individual and your body and brain are not exactly like anyone else's, we might conclude there cannot be a single secret to the golf swing. Similarly, every person has their own ever changing sense of perception or feel.

The great news is that while your sense of feel may vary from day to day, this drill taps into that unique feel for any given day. It also taps into everyone's unique sense of balance and coordination.

It involves how our mind and body's nervous system network optimizes our motor movements and athletic performance. The primary concept of this book does touch on a bit of neuroscience, in fact, but relax, you don't need to be a genius to get the idea or to use it. It is already built into your body and mind system in a way you never thought was possible.

You will be amazed, because much of the power and ability for a great golf swing IS ALREADY WITHIN YOU. In fact the actual learning and performing this golf swing method will not take much time at all, relatively speaking. In addition, it will be ingrained in you almost instantaneously as a new found habit and a well-honed talent that will likely last your entire golfing life.

However, for you to understand why it works so powerfully and with relatively less effort, we should give some background context and explanation. Armed with this deeper knowledge, you will implement it even more effectively with a clearer purpose and intent.

3

Why Is the Golf Swing So Elusive?

We have all the technology and scientific knowledge available to figure out the golf swing, yet nothing seems to work for many of us. The perfect golf swing has indeed become a mystery to most and the holy grail for those seeking to have a swing like the pros.

In the earlier days of the sport we did not have video or even photos to analyze golf swings. Instead what golfers relied upon were principles based on feel, visualization and intent or target. This fact implies that historically, the aesthetics and mechanical perfections of the golf swing held much less importance than actual effectiveness of playing the game well.

One well known expression to sum it up philosophically is that, "You don't want to focus on hitting the ball, you want to focus on hitting your target". That gives a completely different perspective than the modern, mechanical approach of getting your angles perfectly straight, aligning them perfectly, and making the only remaining task, "hitting the ball". If this is your approach, you will indeed hit the ball, but unfortunately it won't go in the direction you wish. Which in golf happens to mean everything.

Mechanically, the golf swing can be a nightmare of complexity. What are the many mechanical issues of the golf swing we must conquer? To start with, there are a multitude of levers, angles, rotations, vectors and planes in the golf swing.

There are other sports with similar motions, but very few have such a long implement as a golf club, such a small effective hitting area as a golf club, such a small ball to hit, and such a variable pattern of shots that can occur, over such long distances, often many hundreds of yards.

It takes sophisticated golf teachers, instructors, coaches and "golf gurus" to help those in search of the perfect golf swing. Many have their own philosophies of how to swing a club and the industry is saturated with tools, aids, and products to help all of the "lost souls" or at least to make a lot of money doing it.

Why do we think we have the solution one day and the next day it disappears, just so we can start over again? The latest hot tip in a magazine or the latest instruction trend can seduce us to believe anything new. Has there been anything really new to learn though? Isn't the game an ancient unchanged one invented centuries ago in Scotland?

A primary problem we must understand is how we try to consciously control our bodily actions to overcome the complexity and intricacy of the golf swing. Unfortunately, sports scientists' studies conclude that our conscious minds' efforts alone, cannot consistently perform athletic motions effectively. Our subconscious minds play a more important role.

What is our most powerful asset that is also the key to solving the golf swing mystery?The human brain, quite frankly. More specifically we may say our subconscious mind. In fact our whole brain and nervous system is more sophisticated than a supercomputer.

It does WHATEVER is needed to accomplish the complicated task of swinging a golf club effectively and consistently. When the subconscious uses it's superpower of balance that has evolved over millions of years, then it is using powers beyond conscious comprehension and on the highest levels of brain and body function.

4

And the Answer Is… Wait, There's More.

T he "Feet-Together" golf drill is perhaps THE best drill ever invented as many golf teaching pros would attest. There may be different names for this drill, but it was allegedly invented sometime in the 1930's. It is based on balance and feel and is simple to explain and execute. It fact, we will not even need photos or illustrations.

How we understand and implement this drill and method will open the door to a lifetime of great golfing. Here is how this feet together, balanced golf drill is done:

Stand with FEET TOGETHER, practically touching, take your golf grip on the club and begin swinging forward and backward in a continuous motion. Swing towards your target and away from it like a pendulum, back and forth.

Arms are extended at the start. The left arm naturally folds as the club swings to the left, the right arm naturally folds when the club swings to the right. Also, the club will naturally arc or wrap around your body slightly, so just let it take it's natural path.

Arms will swing from 6 o'clock to 9 o'clock, or waist high, at first, with relaxed but active arms and hands. IMPORTANT: YOU MUST STAY PERFECTLY BALANCED FROM BEGINNING TO END.

You should have the feel of arms and wrists being free flowing, fairly supple while still actively controlling the club. Feel the natural weight of your arms and the club like a pendulum OR imagine the motion of a swing set going back and forth, without a lot of pushing or pulling.

A natural cocking and uncocking of the wrists is good but not mandatory, as the club head now reaches closer to twelve o'clock both back and through. Your wrists and forearms will also naturally rotate back and through, just let them do so. Depending on your flexibility you can go beyond twelve o'clock to a normal full swing position.

Once again, the CRITICAL element is that you STAY PERFECTLY BALANCED WITH YOUR FEET TOGETHER from beginning to end. This is THE #1 KEY for this drill to work. Do not sway, stumble, or lose balance in any significant way. This includes before during and after the swing, ideally.

It is okay if your knees flex and pump a bit when swinging back and through. This is just your normal, individual way of coping with the weight of gravity and the centrifugal force being created. Allow your hips and torso to turn only as much as needed to support the free swinging arms and club.

You may not realize until you apply this in real time, but essentially this is the model of a perfect swing created in just minutes or less. After you are comfortable in repeating the motion, place a ball in the center of your feet on the ground and hit it with this same exact balanced motion.

The bottom of the arc is always exactly in the middle of your feet or at your sternum. You can place the ball in the center for all irons and fairway woods. For a driver you can place the ball more on the upstroke or towards your front foot if you like.

Just know that if the ball is on the ground, your club must contact the ball just prior to the ground. To do so you must know that the lowest part of the arc is always at the center, regardless of where you prefer to position the ball.

To keep it simple, begin with only a ½ or ¾ swing. When you get accustomed to this swing, you will notice that your shots start more on line, are more accurate and fly straighter with less curve, but ONLY IF YOU REMAIN BALANCED.

Shots will only go about 90% of your full distance because there is less power created when your feet are together. As you get familiar with the motion, then take your normal width stance, but recall the balanced feel when your feet were together.

Now when your feet were together it forced your sense of balance to heighten and activate. You want this feel to remain when you stand in your normal way. With the normal stance you will gain back the 10% of power. You will probably add more with less effort, because your efficiency has greatly increased through the dynamics of a balanced swing.

Even a novice can do this drill very effectively, because even a non-golfer has a finely tuned sense of balance they've been accessing their entire lives. If you are an avid player, haven't played in a while and are feeling,"rusty", then this drill instantly brings your best golf swing back.

It really does, even after long periods of time such as a year or more.

We can see that the golf swing will be created very quickly and simply with this process. The resulting golf swing is highly consistent, predictable, and reliable under pressure.

Let's examine more closely what exactly is going on when we perform this drill. Understanding it better will give us insight and allow us to use it the right way to achieve what we want in the golf swing.

This balanced drill changes every aspect of your golf swing on many levels without you consciously knowing it. The timing of your wrist break, the folding of your elbows and the center positioning of your head and torso are automatically corrected and synchronized. Even your swing plane is corrected as a subconscious reaction to your balanced body position.

In a golf swing, there are about two hundred individual muscles that are being coordinated to make hundreds of microscopic adjustments in a matter of seconds. Therefore, no, you cannot consciously do all of that. It is done mostly subconsciously as long as you make it your central effort to STAY BALANCED THROUGHOUT the swing.

After getting the hang of it you actually won't need to practice your swing as much as you did before. You can essentially have a grooved swing ready whenever you need it. The reason is that this application of balance through activation of our nervous system is highly evolved and hardwired into us, so it is VERY POWERFUL, more than the consciously focused efforts you may have made in the past.

How does this differ from how we more commonly think of swinging

11

the golf club? The overall feeling can be quite different. It will actually feel like more power created with less effort or energy exerted. For example, we do not need to forcefully pull down on the club at the start of the downswing. Instead it's like jumping rope, where we direct the energy inward to the center of the rope handle.

Another factor that effortlessly produces power is that of "double pendulum" levers created by the elbow, wrist and club. This element will exponentially create synchronized power. You don't need to know all the details or physics laws that make it work. Just know that when swinging seamlessly and in balance, this is how efficient rotational velocity is created seemingly without trying.

Another way to describe this balanced swing is as if swinging a weight such as a small rock on the end of a short, 12 inch string, let's say. In order to swing it as fast and smoothly as possible, we would hold the center of the arc, our hand, very still and see how the weight rotates incredibly fast with very little motion of our hand at the center of the rotation. We are effectively creating more speed and more power with less effort.

Not only that, by counterbalancing the weight of our swinging arms and club with our body we will create a more consistent arc, correct swing plane and angle of attack, i.e., the steepness or shallowness of club angle into the ball. We will make more crisp contact and be more accurate with our shots with more power and less effort.

5

How Do the Pros Make It Look So Effortless On TV?

W ell, let's observe some of the best players in the world. Take a close look at a PGA professional's golf swing on television, from a face on view. With what we've discussed so far, what we see makes sense and is quite remarkable. Whether the video is at full speed or slow motion, the balance and centeredness of their motion is very apparent.

Other than their feet, their entire body position throughout the swing and balance-wise, often looks exactly like someone performing the feet-together drill. Whether they learned through countless hours of practice or with a drill like the feet-together drill, the element of balance is present and is a MUST. For most of these great players, they will actually play short wedge shots and pitches with their feet together, because no lateral weight shift is needed to gain additional power.

As an example, a player like Patrick Cantlay, has a swing that has been described by commentators as follows, "He is not pulling forcefully from the top of the swing with his arms, but rather it's an inward, rotational force around his center axis…". This accounts for the smooth, seamless appearance of his golf swing.

This is very much how we described our drill by thinking of a jump rope rotating inward on the rope handle or swinging a weight on a string at high speed with the center remaining still. It is also how most if not all the golf swings of the best players in the world look.

Another player we may note is top ranked player, Scottie Scheffler. He has the odd habit of appearing to stand on his left/front foot only through impact and follow through. His other foot slides together and is almost touching the other. It takes great balance to swing like that, just as it is needed in the feet together drill.

We can very logically conclude that the forces he creates are much like that of the feet-together drill. To swing with most or all of one's weight on the leading foot and sliding the rear foot closer to be practically touching, is essentially the same action used in the feet together drill.

Although not every PGA pro swings in this same fashion, in order for Scheffler to swing this way he MUST REMAIN BALANCED in a similar way as the feet together drill. These examples of great players' swings are real evidence that balance in the way we've described and implemented is a key element of a great golf swing.

6

More Aspects of Why This Works.

Numerous others have spoken of and taught this drill, however, I also want to expound on how there are huge, impactful elements that will move your progress by leaps and bounds.

Can we fully explain why it works so well and produces such universal success? Do we even need to, or is it enough to just know that it works?

Well one way to see it is that evolution explains it. Let's call it "Cave Man" theory. Going back to our earliest days as primates, we have evolved in miraculous ways to ensure our survival to become top of the food chain and the most intelligent creature on the planet. The human brain and nervous system is complex and sophisticated beyond belief, because it has developed and refined itself over millions of years. No supercomputer is anywhere near to matching it.

During these millions of years we have more than just survived as a species. So what has happened in all that time? We've reinvented ourselves, adapted, changed, strategized and refined all in the name of survival and evolution.

To put it into the context of this book, because of our need to survive, we have gained among other highly developed skills the ability to balance while in motion. If we did not develop such skills, then we would not have survived and thrived as a species. Let's not forget that in this way we are also doing the bidding of our genes that serve to propagate to the next generation and beyond.

One particular aspect of our evolution, therefore, leads to one of the most phenomenal skills that we humans possess. That is the seemingly basic skill of balance that we often take for granted. In the context of this book we definitely should NOT, since It is highly evolved and as sophisticated as our brains themselves.

Balance benefits our capacity to develop and refine aspects of our movements and this includes athletic movements. Our ability to balance on our two legs is a key element that allows us to perform a vast number of skills in today's most popular sports. With balance, in the midst of an athletic action, we react, adapt and do whatever our powerful subconscious tells us is necessary.

One of the best applications of this powerful balance skill in sports is for any sport that involves swinging an implement such as a bat, club or racket, and/or a motion involving rotary or rotational body movement. Therefore this includes most if not all major sports: baseball, tennis, golf, hockey, and would also include the motions we make in throwing, running, basketball and boxing.

While engaging in any of these sports, if you stand with your feet close together as in this drill, then you have a very limited amount of stability. In other words if you lean too far in any direction you will lose balance and/ or fall. Therefore, when you swing the golf club in this position, your sense of balance MUST kick in, instinctively. Our highly sophisticated brain and nervous system is activated. It subconsciously controls and coordinates hundreds of muscles and thousands of nerves, all in an instant.

As a result you will actually achieve perfect balance, coordination and timing AUTOMATICALLY in order to remain standing. "Automaticity" is one of the defining characteristics of a true athlete, but that is an entirely separate subject. There are entire books written on this subject, including mine, "HIGH PERFORMANCE SPORT SKILL INSTRUC-TION, TRAINING, AND COACHING, by DDJ PUBLISHING.

The magic of this drill is that you can actually use it in play, and in fact hit some of the most accurate golf shots. You likely will find yourself hitting the most perfect shots that you never thought were possible.

As long as you maintain your balance throughout the swing your phenomenal mind and body system will subconsciously change and improve all the mechanical and sensory, feel aspects of your golf swing. These aspects include rhythm, timing, tempo, swing plane, wrist hinge, wrist lag, rotation of the wrists and forearms, knee flex, hip rotation, angle of attack, consistent arc bottom, follow through, and of course centeredness and balance.

Importantly, I'd point out that the exception or one thing this drill may not correct is your grip and resulting club face angle. A proper functioning grip is essential in golf, therefore you MUST also take the time to learn this correctly.

You can look up how to grip the golf club online, from any basic lesson book or from a teacher or fellow golfer. Without a proper grip, your swing will still be completely sound by using the feet together drill, however your club face may not be square at impact. This will result in directional error, side spin and excessive curving either left or right, because of a closed or open club face in relation to the swing path. Fix the grip and you will fix the direction and excessive curve, since the drill ensures an already perfect swing path.

This balanced swing drill can easily be adapted and applied with very similar results for most if not all sports. Some examples are a tennis serve, a baseball swing or pitch, or a hockey shot.

In fact, if you observe many professional tennis players, such as Raphael Nadal, you will see that his feet are in fact together as he serves the ball. He stays balanced with great results. A hockey player obviously requires balance as they are on ice skates, which further backs up the notion that balance is key.

Now in a sport such as baseball, the pitcher takes a great stride forward which creates extra weight shift and power as does the batter for the same reason. There is an additional element of muscular force being exerted. The additional raw power is beneficial, however it is at the expense of some control if overdone. Even so, as the additional power is gained, the proficient power hitter and pitcher have become quite well balanced notwithstanding such extreme speed, dynamic power and force.

On the other hand, if a baseball pitcher is mostly striving for precision control, they would place more emphasis to remain perfectly balanced throughout. For example a knuckle ball pitcher uses much more finesse than power and therefore would take a more highly balanced approach. He therefore would gain superior control where raw power is not the objective.

7

More Than Words Can Say

Interestingly, as we've alluded to, words cannot easily describe how we maintain our balance. To try to explain would be like explaining how we move our knee and hip joints as we walk on stair steps. We would probably fall down if we consciously thought about it too much. We do it subconsciously as our conscious minds cannot process it easily or rapidly enough. It is almost beyond putting it into words.

Go ahead and try to describe how you maintain your balance and it sounds quite odd. The feeling of your body weight pulls in several directions which is counterbalanced by how you hold or move your arms, hips, shoulders all in perfect synchronization to result in the appearance of being perfectly still. It's extremely abstract for the conscious mind. How would you describe it while trying to instruct someone in performing an athletic motion?

Unfortunately, that is the approach most often taken when instructing how to swing a golf club, or how to throw a ball. We would do much better to feel our own balance than try to recreate it through a mechanical description of how to perform it.

Our ways of teaching ideas in sports are often lost in translation. We lose effectiveness and far too much of our natural instinctive powers when we try to verbalize or over analyze our athletic motions.

Part of the beauty of this feet together drill is that is learned almost completely non verbally, without describing the actual process that only our subconscious brains can perform. I believe this balanced exercise is a prime example if not ultimate proof of our innate physical skills and abilities.

Our potential for learning skills at high levels greatly improves, when we understand how to tap into it. We must use ideas like this balanced drill that are simpler, more goal oriented, and more based on our senses and feel than external instructions.

Drills are the best way to teach natural and athletic movement. They are not a verbalization, but an actual practice of the motion and sensing it within not from someone else's instruction or interpretation.

Your own mind/body, brain/nervous system produces great athletic results if you allow it to. The process and actions are instinctive, even if you are not an avid golfer or athlete. Regardless, you still have access to this tremendous power of balance as you have your entire life. It was hard wired into you from mankind's millions of years of adaptation, the natural laws of survival of the fittest, and evolution.

8

A Rundown of Thoughts and Benefits

Here is a final list of thoughts and some of the benefits of this balanced method and drill. The positives are numerous and can be experienced by the entire golfing population.

Countless numbers of golfers of all levels, experts and coaches are the source of the following bits of wisdom. They are useful to include here without having to meticulously explain them. Just know that they will likely manifest as you continue to apply this powerful, natural learning process and method. In no particular order they are:

If your timing is off and you are mishitting golf shots, you can always come back to this drill.

A helpful thought is that you aren't swinging to stay in balance, but are swinging in balance throughout. That is the goal which creates great results.

Research has been done on this drill. Results have proven that golfers will rotate and turn in a more consistent and centered way. The path of their club will be more consistent as will the bottom of their swing arc and the resulting ball contact.

The knee and head will maintain their levels, thereby creating consistency.

Proper balance builds consistency and control, and that is what is needed in golf at a premium.

Some teaching pros go so far as to say most people should actually play this way with feet together, because it is so much more effective than what they are doing.

It synchronizes the upper and lower body. It brings back your timing if you've lost it.

It stops swaying and stops you spraying the ball in all the wrong directions.

You will know whether you are doing it well, and receive your own feedback by either remaining in balance or stumbling after a swing. When you stay balanced, you start hitting perfect shots.

It is very straightforward and to the point. It encourages freely swinging the arms in rhythm (instead of tensing up to hit the ball forcefully). It also adds the critically important elements of tempo and rhythm.

It is a great, simple drill that self corrects. For example, if your backswing gets a bit flat, this drill helps get the arms 'lifting' up and onto plane rather than swinging around the body at the halfway back point.

The key is balance. You need to maintain balance in order to execute this drill properly, and this balance also fixes a number of faults.

Other swing errors that this simple drill will aid include, swaying on the backswing, over swinging, insufficient wrist hinge on the backswing, starting the downswing with the shoulders and coming over the top and not rotating the forearms through impact.

Many golfers love this drill, because they can actually hit golf balls and see the results. The only downside to playing your round of golf like this are that you do not generate as much power. However, more often than not, the golf ball is hit straighter and more consistently with the feet together than with the feet apart.

Some players use too much body movement. This drill is most effective for them. If the arms get "locked up" to the body with an insufficient swinging action, you lose your balance. Use this drill and you will get a freer arm swing.

9

Conclusion

T he benefits and problems solved solved by this drill are almost infinite. We are all different and have our own individual quirks and faults unique to us. I could list some more types, but suffice it to say that you would be well off to just know that your most critical faults will be addressed by this method.

In a general sense, you may not even need an explanation why it works, but will surely see the results. The answer will lie in your individual relationship with balance. The answer is in how your body and brain have the ability to self correct when using the superpowers of the subconscious. We must give thanks again to the millions of years of humankind's development and refinement.

A note of caution, we humans are extremely resourceful and can find ways around the benefits that this drill gives. So beware that if you stubbornly make an effort to do the wrong things, you may destroy the benefits of this drill.

You must understand what it does for you, which then allows you to create a feedback loop for success in honing your golf swing and playing skills. Understand the overall and the finer aspects of what you are gaining with this drill.

Essentially, dare I say, you are on a path to solving the great mystery of the golf swing for good. This is not a drill that works for just one day and not the next, like many other temporary fixes fallen by the wayside.

One key reason is that while your feel each day may differ, this drill taps into your unique feel for any day. Similarly, as every person has their own sense of feel, it taps into their unique sense of balance and coordination on any given day.

It is a tool for getting you back on track whenever you need it. For example, If you don't know why you are out of sync and don't know what to do, you can use the drill in mid-round to fix your swing. You can also use it as a pre-shot routine. As stated already, you can even play all your shots using this drill.

My hope in writing this book is by sharing my experience and what I've gained from learning this phenomenal drill and method it will help create the basis of your lifelong skill in playing golf. I've been a very skillful, low-handicap player for several decades by working hard at it. However, when I learned this method, I no longer needed to practice very much to maintain or improve my swing.

I've also had this as a go-to, immediate refresher, so I never need to "relearn" or change my golf swing when it's a new season, for example. Since learning and using this drill, I now play better, practice less, truly realize the potential of my golf swing, and therefore love the game that much more.

Many others have professed and praised this drill and method, but few go into the depth of explanation or background I've included in this book. I've tried to impart some of the scientific based as well as the intangible, less common aspects in order to emphasize how truly miraculous this swing method and concept is.

How this method functions so effectively is tied to the miracle of our human body and mind system, so is it really that unrealistic to call it miraculous? This evolved, skill resource has taken a relative "eternity" over eons in it's creation in us humans. Learn and take advantage of it in the right way, and it can last a lifetime.

I hope it helps you create a lifetime of enjoyment of this great game. Enough said, so go out and play golf using this powerful method for success.